DAVID'S JOURNEY WITH SCHIZOPHRENIA

Insight into Recovery

DAVID LaCHAPELLE

.
ISBN: 1500880078
ISBN 13: 9781500880071
Library of Congress Control Number: 2014914887
CreateSpace Independent Publishing Platform
North Charleston, South Carolina

God, grant me the serenity to accept the things I cannot change, the courage to change the things I can, and the wisdom to know the difference.
—Reinhold Niebuhr

CONTENTS

INTRODUCTION

One person in one hundred will develop schizophrenia. You may be suffering from schizophrenia and need some support. Maybe you have a loved one dealing with this condition and want to help, or your profession entails caring for those living with mental health challenges. In any case, you have come to the right place.

During the publication of my first book, *David's Adventure with Schizophrenia: My Road to Recovery*, my editor advised me to integrate my insights into recovery into the work. I did not heed her advice because I wanted the book to focus mostly on the cross-Canada journey I took with my girlfriend at the time and only briefly touch on the events in my recovery. Today, I'm in a more favorable position to reflect on my challenges with the illness.

In *David's Journey with Schizophrenia: Insight into Recovery*, I will take you to the front lines of what it is like to live with schizophrenia. I will share my struggles in coming down with schizophrenia and experiencing undesirable health and life circumstances, moving to a new town and trying to meet new people, attending university after being out for almost seven years, being admitted to the hospital because my medication switches and adjustments were not working, and being employed full-time. I'll detail my insights into the process of finding a good friend, the ups and downs with my medications, and what I have learned from my experiences with spirituality and God.

As a society, we must remove the stigma projected toward those living with mental illness. This book will dispel many of the myths and mysteries about schizophrenia. My fourteen years of experience so far with coping, battling, and perennially conquering this brain disorder will do just that. This irreplaceable experience is worth its weight in gold, and I hope it brings immense value to you.

PART 1:

THE JOURNEY OF RECOVERY

ONE

COMING DOWN WITH SCHIZOPHRENIA

I arrived in Ottawa to attend Carleton University at the age of twenty-three in the autumn of 1996. Ottawa, being the capital of Canada, is the hub of political and federal governmental activity for the land. Canada has two official languages, French and English, and this cannot be more evident than when you visit or live there. Ottawa has a population of roughly a million residents, and this fluctuates when tourists visit and university students exit the town in the summertime.

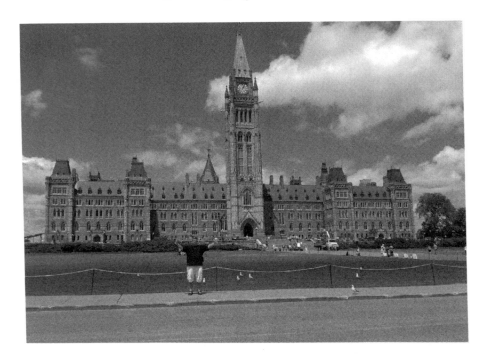

For my first year at Carleton, I was living in residence at Lanark House, on the second floor. Meals were provided in the dining lounge, and there were many restaurants and pubs on campus to suit your fancy if you wanted to eat something other than cafeteria-style food. You could access any building on campus through connecting underground tunnels because of the extreme winter weather.

I enrolled in the political science program, hoping that I would get accepted into the electrical engineering program the following year. All I had to do to qualify was obtain good grades in the preengineering stream: Introduction to Calculus, Algebra, Chemistry, and Physics. I did not fare too well in these courses and continued my post-secondary education with political science and linguistics classes throughout the rest of my two years here.

I did not know what to expect or what I was getting myself into by attending university, but I discovered, to my disappointment, that it was not anything like community college. Because my reading and writing skills were not up to par, I found the workload to be overwhelming. I was used to applying myself in a more practical manner, solving problems with friends or in a group setting. Also, the juggling act between academic studies and socializing was tough.

I found that the students I came in contact with were a few years younger than me, and were experiencing independence for the first time. They were experimenting with different interests and challenges, to develop and discover who they were. That is why most of the students I knew were not serious. Carleton had the lowest entrance percentage grade in the country, but it did offer specialized programs that were pertinent to the technological, political, and journalistic landscape of the city.

Many of my fellow classmates were competitive, superficial, and deceitful. It was a bad scene, as I came from a dysfunctional family environment and lacked awareness about how others from nondysfunctional families lived. I had been kept in the dark about how to prosper in this world, as my parents were not knowledgeable about it and were never on the same page as far as raising a family was concerned.

My mother and father divorced when I was four years old because they could not get along, and infidelity ensued. My mother, younger brother (by one year), and I lived in the suburbs of Toronto until I entered junior high school, and that is when I went to live with my father, who lived in the same city. I chose to live with him because I could not take my mother's mistreatment any longer. I had turned twelve years old, when, by law, I could decide on my own with whom I wanted to live.

While growing up, I never had a good relationship with my brother. Unknown to me, my mother had told him to stay away from me because I was dangerous. My brother was scared of me. I had been treated like a criminal ever since I could remember, and that angered me. I was forced to rebel against the fictitious identity they had created for me, and I became the black sheep of the family. I would take refuge in many friends and their loving families over the years and prayed that one day the tables would turn. In the meantime, I was the target at home as my mother ruthlessly launched her emotional terror campaign at me.

My mother's hypervigilant approach to abusing me was intended to catch me off guard, to rape me of my personal power. She would make demeaning comments to insult me, put me down, and induce guilt, or play devil's advocate to garner a negative emotional response. There was no way to shield myself from this, and I would eventually break down and defend my innocence.

Once I opposed her about her abusiveness, opening the door for her to criticize and belittle me. Then she played the victim when I retaliated with physical outbursts. It was her sole ambition in life to drive me into the ground. Instead of getting love and support from my mother, I got the opposite and never could understand why.

In turn, I had a longing to gain knowledge about myself and to experience the world. I wanted to learn more—to get outside the bubble of Toronto and a dysfunctional family environment—and going to university was my first chance to spread my wings. Then when freedom seemed within reach, I became aware that I was coming down with some kind of mental illness, but I could not accept that there might be something not right with me.

I had too much pride to give in and see a doctor. I attempted to carry on as if everything was fine, as if I could resist God's gentle yet forceful hand. I was aware of the fact that I was falling apart and that the manner in which my personality used to serve me did not work for me anymore. I was lost. I felt love guiding me but had fear of the unknown and of how exactly my life was going to play out. It felt that I was on automatic pilot to destroy everything I knew or was. Being lost was a frightening experience, and I thought, *There must be a way to get off this track.* I looked around for someone to help me, but there was no one. It seemed that I was the only person going through this experience of being paranoid and fearful, and I realized I would have to face my fears on my own.

I was twenty-six years old when I was expelled from Carleton in my third year for violating academic probation for the second time. I was released from my duties at the Brick, a furniture, appliance, and electronic superstore, where I was an office worker, and I gave my notice to my landlord two months in advance that I would be vacating the unit. I decided to move back to Toronto but had no plans to live with my mother and brother, even though they wanted me to.

I lived out of my car for a couple of weeks, until one day I went to my mother's apartment for some food, only to discover that my family had obtained a Form II from the justice of the peace, to have me committed to North York General Hospital. Since my stay at the mental health ward was short, there was no time for the doctors to diagnose me and administer treatment. I had met Angela, a fellow patient in the ward, and hired her attorney to get me released from the hospital.

Ontario law in 1999 stated that I could be held against my will for only a seventy-two-hour period; then, after that, I was free to leave. And that's exactly what I did. Angela and I got together a week and a half later, and we decided to travel to Vancouver and back while we were suffering from our unattended mental illnesses. I wrote about this journey in my first book.

There were moments during our trip when our families were aware of our whereabouts and intervened to get me psychiatric care. I refused treatment for good reason—because they never had my best interests at heart. For my situation to change, the inevitable had to occur: I committed a crime and then had treatment forced upon me so that I would be fit for court proceedings. I received care at the Centre for Addiction and Mental Health (CAMH) in Toronto. This is when I started taking the antipsychotic medication Risperdal and began to enter reality. It was another frightening experience, because I recognized how insignificant and vulnerable I was.

I moved to start a new life with my dad in Lindsay, a small town ninety minutes north of the city. I arrived there one evening in the spring of 2000, and the next morning we made the trip to the local hospital to officially receive my diagnosis. I was in the outreach clinic with my nurse when she informed my dad, "David has schizophrenia."

I felt my confidence shatter, and my industry to be a productive member of society and a worthy human instantly evaporate. *How could this happen to me?* I felt the heavy burden of the label on my shoulders, as I was aware of the stigma associated with the word *schizophrenia.*

When I arrived at home, my initial reaction to being diagnosed with schizophrenia was to freak out and scream, but I controlled myself, even as I swallowed the bitter pill of despair. I felt debilitated because this reality was so overwhelming, and there was so much to learn and such a long way to travel to recover. I understood the enormous amount of courage, determination, strength, and patience it would require, and I wondered, *Is it worth it?* I blamed myself for having a mental illness and for ruining my life. I punched myself in the arm and said, *You idiot, Dave, you really did a number on your life now. It is going to take ten years to get out of this mess.* I realized that I had hit rock bottom.

Then I gathered myself and said to God, *This is all you got? Bring it on.*

$\mathcal{T}$ W O

LIFE AND MENTAL HEALTH

$\mathcal{I}$ had drained my life savings and sold most of my worldly possessions for practically nothing when I began my adventure. My father's income derived from worker's compensation; he had injured his hands through years of service of being an electrician. He had also received an inheritance, which gave us the opportunity to purchase a house in town. The fact that we were living on a fixed income was not noticeable to me, since there were limited entertainment and shopping facilities to enjoy nearby. I felt like an immigrant in a foreign country—I was a city slicker, adapting to depressed-small-town life. I knew right away that I could never fit in, much less be an integral part of the community.

It was very lonely because all I had was my father, who did not know how to have a two-way conversation. I had to listen to him putting down others and spouting his negative perception of life. I am grateful to my father for taking me in and looking after me, but that all came at a high price. He cooked healthy meals, looked after my affairs, and gave what he could, but he is an alcoholic, and his unpredictable moods were almost unbearable. My father was controlling in my early years of recovery. It was his way or nothing, and when I went my way, he would pick on me and insult me until I gave up on my choices. I felt robbed and demeaned, but there was nothing I could do because he masked his desire to control with seemingly good intentions. I felt that what was going on was not right, but he was so calculating and persistent I was no match for him and had to surrender to his will. This affected me negatively in my life for many years after, but it also helped me define who I am by who I do not want to be. Anyhow, my dad and I were fully dependent on each other, and buying the house further solidified our commitment to a town we did not want to live in.

We were content to some extent, in that we had a comfortable and slow-paced lifestyle, which was perfect for the early stages of my recovery. This recovery started with the recognition that I was helpless to improve my situation. I had to face the truth no matter how disturbing and unsettling it was. I was in a deep, dark valley and could not see into the future, although I was aware there was one. That gave me hope, even though I was angry with God. I knew I would get better one day, but when that day would arrive, I was unsure.

The initial onset of recovery constituted an ongoing territorial battle between my medication and the illness. It would take many years for the medication to establish itself, but in the meantime, my brain was fragmented, and my emotions were disturbingly fearful. My dysfunctional thoughts raced through the unstructured maze of my mind with such a fierce momentum I was overwhelmed, distraught, and exhausted. I feared fear itself, and everything and nothing at the same time.

There was a sense of urgency on my part to navigate through this confusion and unearth some sanity. This was difficult to accomplish because the pace at which random thoughts bombarded my mind was exhausting. I was desperate to maintain control over the process by connecting meaningful thoughts. I was searching for the truth, as I recognized that this was the only way to obtain stability. The problem was the majority of my thoughts did not make any sense, and the rest were self-defeating lies that overshadowed the real thoughts.

The chatter in my mind led me around in circles, hijacking and occupying my time and space by keeping me preoccupied with my thoughts. I was not in this world, and you could tell. It felt like a race against time, and there was nothing I could do to extinguish the torment. I had to ride this thing out.

The best weapon in my psychological arsenal was to try not to believe my dysfunctional thoughts and emotions. It was not an easy task, as my thoughts screamed in my head and my emotions resonated throughout my body as they attempted to validate each other's existence. I was aware of this early in my recovery and realized that they were not real, and I tried to separate them. I did not want to think or feel that way and I tried to focus on who I really was and who I could be. In the meantime, I was possessed by schizophrenia's will and had to be subservient to so-called normal people because I felt that they were my gateway to healing.

Through my interactions with others, I thought I was in reality, but I was not, and people could sense that. I felt I was conversing in a normal manner, but unfortunately, I wasn't. I was aware that I had schizophrenia, but at the same time, I was in denial. I was torn and twisted between two worlds, thinking and feeling that others were crazy and I was sane, then vice versa.

I wanted to be in control of my environment so I could protect myself, but others would always surprise me by saying or doing the opposite of what I expected, and I felt threatened. At social gatherings individuals I knew would not say hello to me when I thought they should, and strangers on the street would say hello to me when I was not expecting it. At the grocery store or shopping mall when I thought people should walk around me they would walk into me, and when I thought they were going to walk into me they would walk around me. That is why I found it difficult to let go and allow others to be who they were. I knew others were mirroring back to me my true inner state, and I did not like what I saw, but there was nothing

I could do but remain reserved and withdrawn. I did not want to be hurt, and I feared rejection because somehow I felt responsible for how others were reacting to me, and I did not want to confirm their suspicions that I was the cause of their fear.

I would aggressively examine myself by rehashing my social interactions in my mind and just could not make any sense out of what I had experienced. I was lost but desperately wanted to improve how I presented myself. I was searching for myself in others, and that can be a dangerous thing to do. But I recognized that self-acceptance was the key to recovery, and others were barometers of my progress.

As I got out in the world and got more comfortable with interacting with others who were in a similar position as myself, I recognized there's a social stigma attached to schizophrenia. That impeded my coming out of my protective shell. I was treated with suspicion because there is so much mystery and misunderstanding surrounding the illness. People did not know what to make of me. I refused to believe their stereotypes, or that I was a second-class citizen resigned to a life with no future or hope. I realized that it may take many years to heal and build a life for myself and I was willing to wait for my opportunity. I had no other choice. I was surrounded by hostility on all sides, yet somehow I believed I would win. I used any influence, whether negative or positive, to motivate me to overcome the odds. Nothing was going to stop me, even though I lacked an understanding of the process. I was pioneering my way back to health without the help of anything or anyone, except antipsychotic medications and the guidance and comfort of God.

All I could do was set short-term goals. I realized this was the only way I could move forward with purpose. It was intimidating, but I felt that I had been put in this position to test my faith. It was a humbling experience to be disabled and have to struggle to accomplish seemingly menial tasks. The anticipation of all the steps needed to accomplish a goal would overwhelm me. It would take me days to psych myself up to tackle a duty such as basic grooming, and when the day would arrive, I became very stressed out. Everything seemed like a chore. After I accomplished my goal, I was exhausted, anxiety-ridden, and nervous. Although I was fighting against the current, I was aware that if I did not try, I would submit to defeat. And that was not an option.

$\mathcal{T}$ H R E E

P ETERBOROUGH

$\mathcal{W}$e moved to Peterborough, a thirty- to forty-minute drive from Lindsay, in September 2006. The city has several amenities, yet it still has the feel of a small town. It's known for music and has great local talent to draw from. It is also known as a sports community, as there are many National Hockey League players who were born and raised in Peterborough or had their careers start here with the Peterborough Petes. The surrounding area, Kawartha Lakes, is considered cottage country, well known as a four-season playground containing a variety of lakes connected through the Trent Canal waterway system.

We were moderately familiar with Peterborough because we used to shop there occasionally, and I had attended Fleming College to take a creative writing course. We had hopes that we would have a better life in this community and that maybe one day I would attend Trent University. We settled in a small two-bedroom apartment in the southeastern end of town. It was not the greatest area, but we knew this was only temporary until we got our bearings. We needed to get a feel for the community to determine if we were going to stay there.

Within a week, I registered for an Introductory French course at the local college. I felt a little uncomfortable in this small academic group setting, but nevertheless, everything went well. I had a lab partner, Jose, who was accepting of me. We practiced speaking French to each other, and that helped. It was a structured activity that helped me interact with someone and improve my social skills. I did have strange and paranoid thoughts in class that others knew I had Schizophrenia, but I ignored them and ended up earning a B.

In January 2007, I figured I'd take a leap of faith and continue my education by taking the follow-up Intermediate French class. I was mildly paranoid in the classroom, and this time I could not manage my thoughts anymore and they overtook me. My social graces left a lot to be desired, and some of the young students at Fleming were suspicious of me because I was full of fear; their facial expressions showed mistrust, which made me even more paranoid. I could not handle that, so I dropped the class after the second session and never went back.

While experiencing mental health problems during my six months in Peterborough, I was attempting to be more independent from my father. He responded by being more controlling and emotionally abusive. The struggle between us escalated into an argument one day, and I said I was not going to tolerate his behavior any longer. After our confrontation, I packed my personal belongings and some clothes and took the next bus to Toronto.

My mother was surprised that I had left my father unexpectedly to live with her. I felt that God was guiding me to make this decision, and it felt right, even though I did not understand why. I got along fine with my mother, but I could feel that there was no love for me in her heart. I simply existed, there in her tiny one-bedroom unit in a seniors' building, and after a few months, many of the residents became suspicious of me because I was too young to be allowed to live there full-time.

Big-city life was not for me, and after six months, I caved in and accepted my father and his new fiancée's invitation to live with them. They had purchased a house in the west end of Peterborough that had a basement apartment without a kitchen.

I did not know what to expect because my father had turned his past girlfriends against me. I was hoping he was on his best behavior because he was trying to establish a good impression.

The moment I entered the home, I was welcomed with open arms. I realized early on that my father's fiancée, Nancy, was a good woman, though I did wonder at times why she would want to be with my father. I settled nicely into my new digs and realized that I was starting over again and was at a crossroads. My condition was improving, and I was feeling better. My racing thoughts had slowed down, and I was less fearful and paranoid. I was more aware of myself and had been practicing my social skills with the cashiers at the various stores where I would shop.

One day I approached Nancy and said, "I would like to take psychology at Trent."

She immediately replied, "Go for it, David; you can do it."

Because I so often felt humiliated and stigmatized for having schizophrenia, I saw going to university as a good way to redeem myself. I knew that I was intelligent and would do well if I applied myself. I also knew what it took to succeed at university and was conscious of the fact that if I passed up this opportunity, I would have to live with regret my whole life, and that was something I could not do to myself. I felt that by pursuing a dream that was close to my heart and that was also a respected endeavor, I would gain not only a better understanding of myself and others but also confidence and dignity.

My first day at Trent was nerve-racking. I walked into the main lobby of Otonabee College, which housed the Wenjack Theatre, where my first class, Introduction to Psychology, was to be held. I was self-conscious because I had not been around a group of young people for a long time and felt a little out of place. The auditorium was full, holding about four hundred students, and to my uncomfortable delight, I realized I was one of very few guys there.

If that was not enough to wake me up, I also had to contend with the younger generation. My classmates were tech-savvy and they multitasked between eating, chatting, surfing the Internet, playing video games, and typing lecture notes. *Wow, these individuals are definitely different than me*, I thought, initially resenting them for being who they were, yet, at the same time wanting to be like them. I felt alive around these young people who were clearly excited about their futures.

The school atmosphere was contagious because the majority of the students at Trent were serious students, and I fed off their motivation to succeed. Trent is a quality small school that is student centred. My professors were always available and were the leading experts in their fields. You knew what was expected of you, and you just had to do the work.

Even though I enjoyed Trent, it would take me a couple of days to prepare myself mentally for school. It was difficult to motivate myself, as I was full of fear and anxiety. Before leaving the house, and then in the parking lot once I got to school, I would give myself a little pep talk that everything was going to be okay. I felt helpless, thinking constantly about countless, undesirable hypothetical situations that could occur, fearing that I would not know how to handle them and that it would be discovered that I was mentally ill.

In the classroom, most of my experiences were pleasant and enlightening, although I did have a few moments of shutting down in class because of my paranoia and fear. I would either send a signal of fear by looking over at another classmate, which I perceived would make them suspicious of me, or I would be at peace and content within my mind and emotions, and others would send a signal of fear to me by looking over at me. When either of the cases occurred, I would spiral into a rattled and confused state, rendering me preoccupied and out of tune with my social setting.

When I had more experience attending lectures with success, I was able to recover more quickly from the stress of interacting with others in a social learning environment. Even though I did feel a sense of belonging, I figured I was attending Trent not to win a popularity contest but to earn a degree. By remaining focused on the task at hand, there was no room to worry about how I presented myself or about others' perceptions of me. I would build confidence in myself from one successful social interaction or by earning a good grade. I found that made me a little less self-conscious, and I did not need as much downtime to reflect on my perceived bad experiences, as I knew I was doing the right thing, mistakes and all.

Since I did not know anybody in town except for a few people from the Canadian Mental Health Association (CMHA), I didn't have much of a social life. I used to drive to the local casino to play the slots sometimes, to win money and to get out of the house. One day I told my dad, "I am heading out to Kawartha Downs."

He grumbled at me, "Oh, here we go again."

Well, within the hour, I returned home with a profit of just over a thousand dollars in cash, and I flashed it at him with pride. He was not impressed.

I then made the trip to the local Walmart and bought everything a person would need to be able to live on his own. When I returned home, I loaded everything I had purchased into the garage. My dad gingerly entered and looked at me with a blank expression, like he was trying hard to repress his devastation. I was not even looking at apartments or places to live at the time, but I knew I was moving out soon, so I had decided to invest the money wisely before I spent it on something else or lost it all back at the casino.

A couple of months passed, and during this time period, I was getting pressure from Nancy to find a place of my own. I agreed with her that moving out would be the best thing for me. I am thankful to Nancy for pushing me out of the nest, freeing me from the grasp of my father, who did not want to let me go. Even though I feared the unknown and was overwhelmed by the responsibilities of being independent, I made the decision to call Peterborough Housing and ask them to find me an apartment. I was accepted a couple of weeks later.

It was an unusually warm day when I moved into Anson House on October 1, 2010. The air was calm, with no immediate signs of a chilly autumn breeze. This was a rare occurrence, and it seemed the world had paused for a moment of stillness to recognize my monumental accomplishment. I had mixed feelings about living on my own, as I was about to start a new chapter in my life. I had to welcome the challenge even though it sparked my fear of the unknown. The potential of a bright future motivated me to stretch beyond my comfort zone. This was something I had to do.

The building is a historic mansion that was converted in 2008 into apartments for people with disabilities. It's situated on top of a hill, and tucked away in the north end of town. Saunders Court and Hilliard Park apartments, both low-income complexes, are on the same property, which is well landscaped with many different types of trees, shrubs, and flowers that are supported by big rock slabs used as retaining walls. The front of the building has a circular driveway, and the noise from busy Hilliard Street is somewhat shielded by the quieter Anson Street. Since Anson House is a twenty- to twenty-five-minute walk to any store or amenity, many of the residents socialize in the gazebo on the complex's front lawn.

I spent most of my waking hours socializing in the gazebo. Despite the closeness of the community, the tenants were always struggling and jostling to find fault with one another. I was naive to think that I was immune from the petty squabbles. In time, I realized that I had become immersed in the negativity, and I was forced to withdraw to my apartment to write my first book. Shortly thereafter, I moved out of the building.

$\mathcal{F}$ O U R

Hospital Admission One

$\mathcal{I}$ moved to Saunders Court in April 2012. The movers put all my furniture and belongings into my new apartment within a couple of hours. A minute after I settled in, I turned on the television to see if it worked, My neighbor immediately knocked on the door. He told me my television was too loud and to turn it down. I told him no problem and apologized. The same thing happened the next day. I realized there was definitely something not right with this person. Immediately I faxed a written complaint to the landlord stating that my neighbor was harassing me and his actions were unwarranted.

He would continue bothering me, especially if I had company over. He would tell us to keep it down. I was left with no choice but to call the local police department. They contacted him to tell him that he should expect some kind of noise because he was living in an apartment. He did not disturb me for a week and then went back to his old routine. So I called Peterborough Housing and told them my dilemma, and they told him the same thing the police did. He resumed his behavior a couple days later.

My neighbor had an awful energy about him that would transfer to me when I opened my door. After apologizing, I would come back into my apartment feeling frightened. He made me feel like a criminal. I had no choice but to stop answering the door.

One day, while I was talking with my landlord, Chantel, about my difficulties, I told her I had a check for her to cover my rent increase adjustment. She said she would come over to pick it up. In my quarters, we had a good chat and a few laughs. I mentioned to her that some people did laundry at odd hours, like at midnight or 5:00 a.m. I could hear the machines running through the wall, as my bedroom was beside the laundry room. She promised to put up a notice to tell people to do their laundry at reasonable hours.

The moment the notice went up in both buildings, Saunders Court and Anson House, my neighbor on the other side asked me if I had put the complaint in. I told her that it was just a suggestion, not a complaint. It was kind of obvious that it had come from me because she had witnessed the landlord come into my apartment. She seemed upset, and I did not know why.

Shortly after I talked to my neighbor about my suggestion that people should do laundry at reasonable hours, some of my neighbors started walking up and down the hallway all night long, going back and forth between apartments. It all started at midnight, and I heard one of my neighbors who never did his own laundry doing it then. He loudly and repeatedly banged the dryer door open and shut. I knew right away that he was trying to lure me out of my apartment.

My suspicions were confirmed when I heard my neighbor say to the man doing laundry, "Did he come out of his apartment yet?"

He stayed, doing four loads of laundry late into the night. After he finished his last load, I felt a sense of calm and victory when he retreated back to his apartment. Two hours passed without a noise. Then around 5:00 a.m., I felt an intense evil presence. I felt that my life was in jeopardy. That is when I heard this man's voice out in the hall as he walked toward my door. I immediately called the police. When the police arrived a few moments later, everybody scattered into their apartments, and I felt that evil presence disappear. I felt safe again.

The next night I heard a noise that sounded like someone was using an electric drill in the laundry room. A couple of hours later, I thought someone threw a rock at my patio door, and then I witnessed the neighbor who never does laundry conversing with my other pestering neighbor outside his patio door. These coincidences set me off, and I called the police again. My neighbors could hear me make the 911 distress call and dispersed to their apartments before the police arrived. I called the police again on the seventh day, and that is when they caught on that I had mental health issues and told me I should talk about these problems with my psychiatrist.

Under my psychiatrist's supervision, I had spent a year trying to wean myself from Risperdal. At the time I started having difficulties with my neighbors, I was in the final transition stage of going from 6 mg of Risperdal to 15 mg of Abilify. I had changed medications because I had wanted to try something new and I was sick of the side effects of Risperdal: increased appetite, lack of motivation, weight gain, anxiety, and sexual dysfunction, to name just a few. However, it was clear from my difficulties with my neighbors, that only taking Abilify wasn't working. We were aware there was going to be an adjustment period for Abilify to work.

While this was all going on, I was trying to distance myself from my family. It was Easter time, and my uncle was coming to visit for the holiday, so my father wanted me to be there. But my family would not talk to me at holiday gatherings. It was like I did not even exist. My father did not help matters, either, because he drove a wedge between family members with his negative gossip.

I tried to ignore my father's phone calls. He assumed that I was not answering the phone because I was sick. But I simply did not want to attend Easter at my aunt's place. He was persistent, calling numerous times, not acknowledging my initial decision to not go. I didn't need the stress of being pressured to attend an Easter dinner I had no intentions of attending. I was in contact by phone with Nancy throughout my whole nine-day ordeal with my neighbors and father. Nevertheless, it was my father who called the police on me.

When the officers arrived, I did not answer the door. Unknown to me, two of Peterborough's finest were ready to help me. I considered it an unnecessary power move by my father, even though I needed an intervention. The police tried to open my window, but it was locked. They then knocked on my door again and told me my dad was not there with them. I answered the door.

They asked me, "What is going on, David? Your dad is concerned."

I told them, "I am having trouble with my neighbors and not feeling too well."

They said, "Would you like to go to the hospital? We will call you an ambulance."

I said, "Sure."

The police led me outside, where an ambulance was waiting for me. I saw my father down the hill in the visitors' parking lot, venturing toward us, and I told the police officers to not allow him to come up—I did not want to see him. The officers followed my instructions, and I entered the ambulance with the help of the paramedics.

I arrived at Peterborough Regional Health Centre in the early afternoon on Easter Sunday. After waiting for a few minutes in the emergency corridor with the paramedic who had checked my vital signs in the back of the ambulance, I was directed down the hall to register my health card with the hospital. Then a nurse escorted me to the crisis unit: a contained area that looked like the rest of the hospital except for four or five cells with bubble windows. I thought, *Wow, this must be a place where everybody is supposed to flip out*, and felt degraded.

I waited on a seat in the entrance for fifteen minutes. The nurses largely ignored me as they stayed in their protected station, though I was given a glass of water. Then a nurse told me that a medical doctor would see me in the interview room. The room had three cushioned chairs that had weights on them so you could not lift them off the floor. It was difficult to keep my voice low because the room had an echo that was meant to disturb any-body who was normal because it was so loud.

The doctor asked me what was going on, and I told him the story, that I was having trouble with my neighbors. His questions were direct and intended to prod me to open up. I elaborated on what I thought I was experiencing and why, and the doctor lis-tened. He then went into the nurses' station, and I went back to sit in my chair. That is when I heard the doctor, through the Plexiglas window, speak in a tone of disgust to the nurses that I had no in-sight into my condition or state of mind. I felt terrible.

Then, a psychiatrist briefly interviewed me. I told him that I was having difficulties with my neighbors and was experiencing fear and paranoia. I waited another thirty minutes, and then a young intern interviewed me. This psychiatrist-to-be was a young man who looked like he had everything going for him.

He asked me, "What is going on, David, and how did you get here?"

I told him the story of my interactions with my neighbors and my dad calling the police. He then asked me general questions, such as when was I born, what is the date today, and who is the prime minister of Canada. I answered all his questions quickly and correctly, and he told me he did not see anything wrong and that everything seemed to be okay.

He came back a few moments later and asked if I had commu-nicated with any support network throughout this ordeal. I told him that I had been conversing with Nancy by phone and that he should talk to her.

He asked me, "What would you like to come out of this experience?"

I told him, "I would like to get the stamp of approval that I am fine, and for you to let me go."

A few moments later, he came back and said that I could vol-unteer to stay at a hospital, or if I refused, he was going to hold me against my will. Either way, I was being committed. He told me there was no room in Peterborough and that he would transfer me to Ross Memorial Hospital in Lindsay.

I told him, "I am not going to Lindsay. You will find an opening for me here, and I look forward to staying in Peterborough."

I was given a cell, and the door was left unlocked so I could use the washroom around the corner. I lay down on the cot to rest and was only in the cell for a minute when a nurse arrived and asked me if I would like a meat sandwich.

I asked her, "What kind of meat is in the sandwich?" She said she was not sure. I thought to myself, *Wow, should I take the chance and eat the mystery meat or starve to death?* I ate the sandwich and discovered that it was minced chicken. It was gross.

I waited in this transition area for three days, and then on the third day, I was told a room was available upstairs. A nurse escorted me to the locked adult inpatient unit that was for people who were not in crisis. I arrived at night, so I settled in and tried to go to sleep, but I couldn't relax because it was hot in the room and that made my roommate toss and turn in his bed all night.

The next day I asked for a room transfer, and it was approved. I had a double room all to myself for a few days, until my new roommate, Daniel, arrived. I did not know what to make of him at first, but something told me to try to be friends with him. He seemed like a nice guy, but at times he was indifferent. I thought he probably had just come down with schizophrenia and was having mixed emotions. I understood his pain and confusion and wanted to help him.

I spoke to his father in the hallway and shed a few tears as I said to him, "Do not let him out until he gets stabilized, because he will run away." Then my suspicions were confirmed when he left a note on my table stating that he was going to take off to Toronto. But he was unable to check himself out of the mental health ward.

I told Daniel I had written a book, and he thought that was pretty cool. I then signed a copy for him as a gift. I was kind of pushy with telling him that I had schizophrenia because I wanted to help him so much. I knew he was angry, and I think he just wanted to figure things out on his own. He then transferred to a single room down the hallway, and he left the book I gave him in my room. I felt rejected but understood that what I was subtly trying to say to him—that he may have schizophrenia—was difficult to digest.

Twice a week, usually in the mornings, cute female student nurses came into the ward. They would check my blood pressure and ask me if I had a bowel movement the day before. I would always tell them I had, and my blood pressure was always good. It took me about a week to get involved in the mental health ward's programs, such as going for walks around the hospital and attending and contributing to psychoanalysis therapy classes every weekday. The ward psychologist instructed me to be involved in the activities and to take day passes. Overnight or weekend passes would also help with my recovery and being independent.

During my stay at the mental health ward, my psychiatrist gradually increased my dose of Abilify to 30 mg, which was 15 mg more than I had been taking before. He also added 1 mg of Risperdal. I was released after being there for three weeks. I was glad to leave but also a little concerned with how my neighbors would react to me having been in the hospital. When I came home, though, most people said they had been concerned about me and were happy to have me back, even though the only two people who came to visit me at the mental health ward were Nancy and my father.

$\mathcal{F}$ I V E

HOSPITAL ADMISSION TWO

When I got released from Peterborough Regional Health Centre mental health ward in the spring of 2013, I was doing quite well. Not only had I quit smoking, but I was also very active, riding my electric bicycle around town, running errands and enjoying the weather. I also started taking the bus by myself and didn't feel as paranoid in the close quarters of public transit. I would shop at the local grocery stores and hang out on the patio at a local pub to play free poker with my friends.

I was more independent than ever before until my e-bike broke down and I had to rely solely on Peterborough transit. At the time, because I was feeling better, my father and I came to a mutual agreement for him to lend me his car. I would drive out of town to visit Nancy, who lived a few hours away, and to visit my new friend Joe, who had a trailer overlooking a lake. Getting out of town allowed me to see different parts of the country and do some writing.

Abilify seemed to work throughout the summer, although it was not as reliable as Risperdal. I could still function relatively well despite feeling a bit "off." The main noticeable difference was I felt okay when I was active, but the moment I laid my head down to sleep, I would feel weird, as if I should not be resting.

Then one day in the early fall, I broke down in the psychiatrist's office over the suffering I had endured in all those years of dealing with schizophrenia. I had put on a brave face for so many years, and this was my chance to let it all out. I then explained to my psychiatrist that I had felt great for most of the summer but kept to myself that this newfound reality—that there are so many selfish people and that the world can be cruel—was overwhelming and had set me back emotionally. I had been doped up on Risperdal for almost thirteen years, and my eyes were open for the first time. The process of digesting this new perspective may have affected my mood somewhat. Nevertheless, my psychiatrist suggested that I should get rid of the 1 mg of Risperdal. But she quickly retracted her statement, saying that she had made a mistake and I in fact needed to be on Risperdal.

I hated Risperdal because of its terrible side effects and looked forward to getting the drug completely out of my system. Even though the doctor did not want me to discontinue the drug, the seed of being rid of Risperdal had been planted in my head. When I got home that night, I stopped taking Risperdal and felt great. After three days of being Risperdal-free, I was fine. Then, on the fourth day, I realized I needed to be back on Risperdal, but it was too late. Abilify was just not powerful enough to take care of business on its own even though I was on the maximum dosage of 30 mg. I wanted Abilify to work so badly, and so I stayed with it as long as I could even though it was too unstable.

I spiraled down quickly into a functioning state of psychosis, and it seemed my neighbors were concerned about me because I was so quiet in my apartment. First I heard an electric scooter in the hallway by my apartment door that sounded like the one that belonged to a particular person I knew over at the other building. I heard some of my other neighbors, too. They were trying to get my attention by knocking on my door. Then my suspicions were confirmed when I heard this person cough repeatedly—he is a heavy smoker—and they told him to keep it quiet.

That day, after everyone finally left, I decided to drive around town, getting random directions from the voices in my head, with no particular concrete destination. I ended up at a downtown park. I sat in my car in the parking lot, where it was chilly and raining. I parked the car, turned up the stereo to my MercyMe CD, and started to cry profusely. I thought the more I cried, the more power I would have over evil people. I would be healed—free. I eventually made it back to my apartment, taking the long way home, following the directions from the voices in my head.

I arrived at my apartment around 6:30 p.m. and prepared to settle in for the evening. Then, around 11:00 p.m., I heard two men listening at my door. It seemed they were attempting to pick my lock to get into my apartment. While these two guys were at my door, someone tried to open my bedroom window from the outside, but it was locked. I was lying in bed, immersed in a state of psychosis.

I thought, *If those two guys get into your apartment, you're a dead man. You can't defend yourself, and if this is how God wants to end your life, then you must be prepared to die.* Then, while I was wrestling with my fears in this precarious state of mind, I had an epiphany that I was probably sick and that all the delusions I was having were probably not true. This was a big step for me: to recognize, in the midst of my suffering, that my mental health was in question. I fell fast asleep.

The next morning, I woke up and realized that something had to change and that I couldn't go on like this. I drove to the nearby convenience store and bought some cigarettes. I reasoned with myself that it was getting expensive to shop so much, and that I had more than I ever needed. I had been everywhere, and there were no more places to go. Then, out of nowhere, I experienced a restless feeling and felt that I did not belong in society. I then felt pressure from a spiritual force and the outside world, guiding me to the hospital. I did not fight this force and drove directly to Peterborough Regional Health Centre.

Strangely enough, as I was being admitted to receive care, there were my father and brother in the emergency department, escorting my dad's new fiancée Betty because she had fainted at home. There went my plan to seek help anonymously.

I didn't have to wait too long to enter the crisis unit. After a short time, a medical doctor interviewed me—the same doctor who had interviewed me the first time I went to the mental health ward. He told me he was happy to see me, and was impressed at the insight I had into my condition.

After a few minutes, another psychiatrist interviewed me. I told him that I was hallucinating and having trouble with my neighbors again. I told him I had stopped taking the 1 mg of Risperdal and that I felt sick. I felt like a rock star when he told the nurses that I wrote a book and that my mood was always good. The psychiatrist was the same doctor who had cared for me the first time I was admitted, and he knew of my situation with my family and neighbors.

After the nurses and my psychiatrist collaborated on what to do with me, one of the nurses came out from her station and in-formed me that the doctor would like to admit me for a few days and, if there was anything I needed to pick up at home, I should go and get it now. So I drove back to my apartment and got some of my clothes, instant coffee, a few books, an MP3 player, and hy-giene items. I parked my car at the Peterborough Regional Health Centre lot not knowing how much it might cost me, but I was pretty sure they gave leniency to those who were admitted to the hospital.

In the crisis unit, I met a man named George. He said he was having a nervous breakdown and his life was in disarray, so he had decided to seek some help. We were admitted at the same time, and after we had a cigarette together, we were escorted to the mental health inpatient ward. George had been getting impatient with having to wait so long to get admitted. When George and I were getting transferred to the inpatient unit, one of the security guards made a derogatory comment about us to the nurse—that he was embarrassed to escort such a sad bunch or something to that effect. I brushed off the comment and reasoned with myself that I needed help and that I had come to the right place to get it, so nothing else mattered.

As I waited in the television lounge for my room to be assigned to me, I noticed Ruth, a familiar face from the last time I was in the hospital. She smiled at me, but looked embarrassed to be in the mental health ward again. I waited a couple of hours before anyone even acknowledged my existence. Then a nurse came out of the station to see me and pretended she did not know that no one had designated me a room yet. I thought there was a passive-aggressive nature to her behavior and wondered if a guy could get a break once in a while from always being mistreated.

Anyhow, when I did get my room, there was a young man in his early twenties sleeping there, and for three or four days, sleep was all he did. His name was Donny, and once I got to know him, and got past his quiet and reserved demeanor, I learned he was a good guy who had made some bad decisions in his life and was experiencing the difficulties that came with drug addiction.

Donny cracked me up one day, when I asked him in the hallway, where he had stationed his mini home stereo for everybody to enjoy, what kind of music he was listening to. He told me he was listening to the oldies. I knew what I was listening to was retro, but when Donny said *the oldies*, I started to laugh and told him now I knew how old I was. It was clear to me that the music was from the eighties, but I guess I never realized how old I was and how time had passed me by. Donny then told me that I had the best laugh he had ever heard. I thanked him for his compliment and continued laughing.

During my stay at the mental health ward, my eyes were glued to the television, which was rare for me because I usually do not watch TV. Anyhow, I was interested in the media attention focused on Rob Ford, mayor of Toronto, and on the many challengers trying to usurp him. I thought this was a clear example of the war between good and evil, and that Rob Ford represented the good in the world. I also enjoyed the entertainment surrounding this political figure who seemed to have no reservations about expressing himself—much to his own dismay. I was convinced that the circus performers trying to shred his reputation were, in fact, evil because I could see their dilated pupils showing more black than normal, evidence that their true colors were shining through the windows of their souls.

My preoccupation with Toronto politics began to fade as my medication started to work. I was faced with a new challenge, as there was a young man in his early twenties who was a Satan worshipper and read *The Satanic Bible* and played wicked music on Donny's stereo. I tried not to be disturbed, but I realized that I was being drawn into a spiritual battle and there could be only one winner. In my mind, I was under attack. I began to feel his strong evil presence and his attempts to instill fear and guilt in me to control me, to draw me away from God. I was well aware of the devil's tactics and realized that this was war. I asked the Holy Spirit to intervene. I began reading the Psalms of David and defeated the formidable foe. In an act of surrender, this young man came to me in hope of reconciliation. I was careful around him because I did not trust him, and then I launched my final assault. As I shed a tear, I asked him if he would like to give his life to Jesus Christ in an act of love, hoping to save the young man from eternal damnation. But he just rolled his eyes.

The patients in our ward were not a lively bunch, and George, who had been diagnosed with bipolar disorder and now just wanted to get the heck out of there, was getting restless. George just wanted to move on with his life, but they were keeping him there to bring down his mania and get him to settle down. In order to do this, they had to find the right medication and dosage level, which would take a little while—at least longer than it took for me to get stabilized on my new medications of 180 mg of Zeldox and 1 mg of Risperdal.

Then Murphy showed up. He was an outgoing, honest, and caring man in his early sixties. We believed he was having early dementia, and he wanted to get the heck out of there as soon as he was well. Murphy told me he watched the American news and the Canadian news and that was all he asked for—to be able to watch the news. I told him that he would have to tell other people about his wishes, because I was not in control of everything.

One day we went for our walk around the hospital's grounds to get some exercise and fresh air. Before the walk, I had jokingly told everybody to scatter, and told Murphy to take off and make sure to call a cab for himself. Well, even though I was obviously joking, Murphy must have taken me seriously. When we were halfway through our walk and passing by a public school, Murphy ran through the field and took off. He might have slipped away undetected, except another patient noticed him and told the nurse that Murphy had escaped. We sent George, the most athletic person in the group, to run to retrieve Murphy, but he couldn't find him. Then I noticed Murphy standing in the school's entrance, hiding, trying to evade our detection. I told the nurse, and she rounded him up, but Murphy still was determined to get away despite being visually impaired. He ended up breaking free from the nurse and knocked on the door of a neighboring house. He must have showed his "visual impaired" card from CNIB, the Canadian National Institute for the Blind, to get into the home. We did not want any more trouble, so we pretended we were not connected with him.

Then, as the nurse was informing the hospital that Murphy had strayed, a taxi entered the driveway of the home that Murphy was in, and he took off in the cab. The nurse immediately called the police and the taxi company on her cell phone just down the street from where Murphy was and had Murphy intercepted on his way to Port Hope, a town an hour away. He was brought back to the hospital, where he stayed in the crisis unit for a night.

When Murphy was brought into our ward the next day, we all laughed. The big joke in the ward was "Anyone need a cab? Anyone call a cab lately?" I laughed with Murphy, and seemingly, he took the brunt of our jokes with good humor.

It was Christmastime, and the student nurses, with help from a few patients, decorated the ward and its two Christmas trees. In therapy class, there was one social worker in particular who tried to be funny, and the head nurse felt he was a special person, so I convinced the student nurses to decorate the entrance of his office door with lights. When I was leaving the ward after staying there for two weeks, I told the social worker that he must be special to have his door decorated, and he smiled at me, not knowing that I was the guy who had brought it to reality.

S I X

WORKING

$\mathcal{A}$ couple of weeks after getting out of the hospital, I decided to attend Christmas 2013 dinner at my aunt's place. Unfortunately, going there turned out to be a big mistake because I was ignored the whole time I was there. I thought maybe the family had changed, but I discovered that they were all the same as before. My father and his fiancée Betty came to my place a couple weeks later to visit, and ignored me the whole time. It was like I wasn't even there as they talked to each other in front of me. After my father and his girlfriend left my place, I decided that I had had enough. I wrote my family off and changed my telephone numbers.

I was lonely, having only Nancy to talk to over the phone. So I decided to join the Canadian Mental Health Association volleyball club again, which met on Thursdays at the local YMCA. At the same time, I began attending the church down the street from me and I enjoyed worshipping the Lord with other believers. They had a band with singers, and those in attendance sang along, following the lyrics posted on two big projection screens.

But volleyball and church activities were limited, only twice weekly, and I spent the rest of my time all by myself in my apartment. When I visited my psychiatrist in March 2014, I told her that

I needed a job. She told me to go to the Canadian Mental Health Association employment program and ask them what they had for me or if they knew of someone who was hiring. Immediately after my doctor's appointment, I went to CMHA, and the woman at the employment centre asked me what area of work I was looking for. I replied, "Anything," and then got a little more specific, saying that I was looking for a tech-related job. She then stated that there was a company in town that was having a job fair. I thought that I had already applied at this company the previous year and no one had called me back, but I was willing to give it another try. Anyhow, when I returned home, I applied online for a technical customer service representative position.

I stopped going to volleyball and church because it seemed that I could not meet anybody to socialize with. Around this time, I suddenly came down with a really bad cold. I thought I could fight it on my own, but I did not realize that the cold had turned into pneumonia. At the point when I actually fell to my knees coughing, I realized that I needed to go to the hospital, but I didn't feel like calling an ambulance. There was no way I could drive there, so I broke the pact that I had made with myself and called my father.

My father arrived at my place within forty-five minutes and took me to the emergency department at the Peterborough Regional Health Centre. We waited over four hours to see a doctor, and when I did see him, he gave me a prescription for antibiotics and some asthma inhalers. My dad and the rest of my family were glad to have me back again, and after a couple of weeks, my father gave me some money to sign up for an online course to get a security guard license to practice in the province of Ontario. The online security course was not what I thought it would be, and I became disillusioned and disinterested. I got frightened at the mention of security officers who did not follow proper procedure and ended up getting hurt.

Almost two months after I applied for the technical customer service representative job, I got a phone call from the company asking me if I was still interested in the job. They asked me to come in for an interview. I had totally forgotten that I had applied for that job and was caught off guard when I received the phone call. I did my research on the company before going to the interview and Googled interview questions that I might encounter, to be prepared. I knew the company was all about teamwork, so I was ready to state that I was a team player before they even asked.

In the interview session, two people from the company took turns asking me questions. First they asked: *What was a bad job experience that you've had, and what was a good one?* To answer the first part, I told them about an experience I'd had when I'd installed Interac machines in the greater Toronto area. Once I had a customer who insisted on getting an accessory from my old employer. I was supposed to deliver it, but my old employer wouldn't give me that product. My customer was mad when I arrived without the accessory. Then, for the good experience, I told them about a customer who was running a Subway restaurant. After I completed the job, he was so pleased he said I could have anything I wanted from the menu, so I ordered two subs and two chocolate milks.

The interview went smoothly, and Human Resources asked me if I was a team player, and I stated that I was. They were also impressed that I was able to navigate through the insane Toronto traffic to get from one client to another.

I got the job and filled out the paperwork just a week and a half later. I started my training in June 2014. It was scary at first because I was in a room with about twenty other strangers, but after the training session, we bonded and became like family. The training consisted of getting familiar with Apple products and the technical issues that may arise for our potential customers. We trained on the Mac mini, and I learned about Apple devices and became familiar with Apple itself. We learned the soft skills necessary to bring a positive experience to our customers who were calling in for our help or guidance. We learned how to deal effectively with the different types of customers we might encounter.

We were given ten-minute breaks every hour and a thirty-minute lunch. Our assigned trainer was positive and motivational, and high-fived us when we left for the day. We had "clapping wars" with the training class in the next room.

I had training classes from 9:00 a.m. to 5:00 p.m. for four weeks. Then, when I trained in the call centre, taking calls with the help of supervisors or floor support—the shift was 1:00 p.m. to 9:30 p.m. for one week; then 12:30 p.m. to 9:00 p.m for one week. The next week after that it was 10:00 a.m. to 6:30 p.m.; then the week after that my shift was noon to 8:30 p.m. Being on different shifts meant I had to take my medicine at different times, and my morning routine that I was so used to in classroom training was gone. When I got home from my 8:30 p.m., 9:00 p.m., or 9:30 p.m. shift, it would take me a few hours to wind down, eat dinner, and take my pills.

I lived on pins and needles and in suspense every day at work, wondering when would I get a call, what would the calls be like, would I be able to understand the customers, and what kind of problem would they present to me to fix. I found it difficult to hear the customers because the sound quality was not good on my headphones, and it was loud in the call centre because of the other agents taking calls. I always had to have the customers spell their names, and then I'd get their telephone numbers and serial numbers of the products they were calling in about. If I got that far, then I would be able to see if the customers had a warranty or not. If the customers were out of warranty, then I would have to sell them one in order to help them. I had to log the case notes and classify customer issues on the computer while I was talking to them. When I had a complex issue I could not solve, or the customers needed to be transferred to a different department, I would send them to a senior adviser or to the appropriate department.

My first memorable customer was a lady who said to me, "Can you see how beautiful I am?" I told her my computer screen was glowing with her beauty. Then the next week, without floor support, I advised a customer that he was out of warranty, and I sold him an exception, having no clue how to solve his problem or if I could solve it at all. I solved the customer's Wi-Fi issues by getting him to turn off and on his iPad. Immediately, when the customer told me I fixed his issue, I started cheering, and my coworkers all watched me with intrigue.

But it wasn't always this smooth. Some customers' devices couldn't connect to iTunes. I would never know how to solve this issue and became stressed out trying to scramble by asking my coworkers or looking up Apple research articles to try to find a solution to the problem.

The stress from angry customers, changing shifts, and complex problems was too much for me. When I had an angry customer, I would get rattled and feel offended at the ignorance of some people. I was trying my best to help my customers, but it seemed that when dealing with the world, you get all kinds of people. I had one customer who used profanity against me the whole time I was helping him. I found that difficult to digest because I would never be that way to anybody no matter how I was treated.

The stress from the job and the fact that I had changing shifts began to catch up with me. I called in sick one day because I woke up in the morning feeling really ill. I felt overwhelmed, nervous, and anxious. I felt foggy in my mind. I was not myself, and I knew it was only a matter of time and I would become psychotic.

At the workplace, I would usually count the minutes to my first break, then to lunch, then to my second break, and then finally to when I could get the heck out of there. I thought I could hang in there because I liked to socialize with my coworkers and enjoyed having a steady income, but I realized when I took my second sick day to visit my psychiatrist, everything had changed.

I had postponed my doctor's appointment a month earlier because I could not get time off work, so it had been nearly four months since I had seen her last. When I arrived at my doctor's office, she asked me why I had postponed my appointment with her, and I told her that I was working full-time. My doctor was shocked that I had been working full-time for seven weeks. She seemed concerned and asked me if I was getting along with my coworkers, and I told her we loved each other and were like a big family. She then asked if I slept a lot on my days off, and I told her there were a couple of days where I was exhausted, but for the most part, I would clean my house, do laundry, and grocery shop on my days off. I told her that if I felt I had to quit, I would. My doctor then told me she would see me in three months.

I went to work the next day realizing that I couldn't go on like this. The next morning, I had to go to work, but instead I called Human Resources and resigned. The lady that I talked to was disappointed, but she wished me the all the best in life.

$\mathcal{P}$ A R T 2:

Insight into Recovery

S E V E N

FINDING A GOOD FRIEND

S ince I started showing symptoms of schizophrenia, I've been afraid to get out into the world and socialize. Usually, when I would leave the house, I would hope that I would not run into anybody on the way. My goal was an error-free journey. Dealing with other people I came across in my daily life never went smoothly for me because of my mixed emotions and paranoid thoughts. I never got into any trouble, but it seemed that everybody wanted to make trouble with me—or, at least, that's how I felt. I was caught between two mental states: wanting to be left alone, and craving approval from others that I was okay and a good human being.

When I would walk down the street, there would always seem to be somebody nearby who felt uncomfortable in my presence. That would upset me because I just wanted to be accepted for who I was. Even though I realized the problem was mine, I still blamed others for making me feel invalidated as a human being. I learned to live in this unstable state of mind, feeling hurt and incomplete for many years.

When I would drive my car, I was not cognizant of the fact that I had to share the road with drivers who, for the most part, were far more aggressive than me. Vehicles would ride my rear bumper and try to intimidate me to move faster or to get me to do what they wanted. I took it personally. Every time this would occur, I would feel pain in my gut, fear in my heart, and my thoughts would begin to race once again: I felt I was being rejected as a human being.

When I would shop at the local stores in town, I would usually doubt myself about if I should talk to a cashier or not. I lacked confidence and always wondered if I was coming across the right way. I was always second-guessing myself, and this made me feel uncomfortable sharing space with strangers because this affected my delivery and I would be awkward in interacting with others. I was conscious of this relationship, and that bothered me. It seemed that others were aware of my torn self. There was nothing I could do to change how I felt around others, and I wondered if my condition would ever improve.

Then I moved into Anson House in 2010, and I began to associate with the residents in the building. After being isolated for six years in a small town, it was nice to socialize again. I tried to spend time with my neighbors, and stay on good terms, with almost everybody in the building. I was looking for a good friend and naively hoped that by networking, I would find someone I could relate to. Most people in the building liked me, but I found I got caught in the negativity and petty differences the tenants had with each other. I did my best to take the high road, but I discovered that I was on a different level of understanding than these individuals and had to move on in life.

I realized that I needed to downsize my social circle to one person, and sought the friendship of someone who I thought was decent and normal. Pat also lived in Anson House, and he and I were close friends for a couple of years. I enjoyed his pleasant demeanor and positive outlook on life. Pat enjoyed quiet times and his own company just as much as I did, and we got along fine. I introduced him to betting on sports legally through our Ontario Lottery and Gaming Corporation and helped him out with using his Windows computer. Our biggest pastime was going to the many coffee shops in town and checking out the scenery of Peterborough. Pat loved to eat, so we would go out to restaurants, or I would cook him a good meal now and then. Pat was a musician and a dreamer, and we talked about how we were going to write and produce hit songs by digitally mastering them over the computer with music production software. That dream, along with his many others, never went anywhere. Pat still writes music, though, so I am hoping he has not given up on his dream. Pat and I parted company after I realized that he was a bit too selfish, secretive, and shady to be a friend I could trust. He would never do anything I wanted to do and I caught him lying to me on numerous occasions.

Then I met a friend, Gilbert, who also used to live in Anson House. Gilbert used to own and manage an office supply business before he became visually impaired. We had a lot in common because we were both suffering from a mental illness and had experienced trauma. I tried to be a good friend to Gilbert, but Gilbert is an agnostic, and I believe in God, so we disagreed many times. Gilbert taught me how to play poker and introduced me to his friends. Gilbert confided in me that he was associating with people he would not normally know with because of his disability. I tried to be the best friend I could be for Gilbert, but I couldn't handle the crowd he hung around with, so I moved on.

Daniel called me up one day and asked me if I would like to go out for lunch. Daniel was my roommate the first time I was in the hospital, and we became good friends during the summer of 2013. We went on a trip to visit Nancy and Wasaga Beach; then a month later, we went to Ottawa. In the fall, Daniel went backpacking across Europe, and when he came back to Peterborough, his job was not there for him. He got a job pretty quickly, though, one closer to his family, so I do not see him that much because he lives and works out of the greater Peterborough area. But he is there for me, and we always have a good laugh when talking to each other about our adventures in this world. Daniel is a civil engineer, and we are both on the same level professionally and personally. It's nice to have a good friend after so many years of looking for one.

$\mathcal{E}$ I G H T

MEDICATIONS

$\mathcal{F}$rom 2000 to 2006, I was taking two medications: 6 mg of Risperdal and 1 mg of Cogentin. I would take them both at bedtime. Risperdal was a newer main atypical antipsychotic drug, but Cogentin was used to stop tremors of the body that older antipsychotic drugs sometimes induced. I do not know why I was on Cogentin for six years because I never had tremors, just anxiety.

The moment I started taking Risperdal, I felt terrible. It was hard to tell at times which was worse, the illness itself or the side effects from the medication, such as lack of motivation, increased appetite, weight gain, constipation, sexual dysfunction, and anxiety. The medication affected me negatively in so many ways I had no confidence in myself whatsoever. I gained about one hundred pounds, going from two hundred to three hundred pounds in a few months. I was full of fear and anxiety, so I was always restless in social situations and afraid to venture into unfamiliar places and meet new people. I could not motivate myself to do anything. When I would take a shower, I had to rush like an Olympic athlete to speed up the signals in my brain just to be able to complete the task in slow motion. I had to psych myself up to do anything because I was so overwhelmed and afraid.

Cogentin blurred my vision and made me sleep a lot in combination with the drowsiness-inducing effects of Risperdal. When I took my medications, I would normally go to sleep within the hour. But if I took my medications and stayed up, I would feel very drowsy but it was difficult to go to sleep because the medications would hype me up after I got through the drowsy stage. My sleep patterns were disturbed, and even though I slept a lot, it felt like there was a war going in my head because of the conflict between the sedative and hyperactivity effects of the drugs. They worked against each other.

From 2006 to 2012, I was on Risperdal but without the Cogentin. In 2006, I became Cogentin-free, and it took a couple of months for my vision to clear. In 2008, I had the Risperdal reduced to 4 mg over a few months because I could not respond to people's social cues; the Risperdal drastically reduced the dopamine levels in my brain. Once I stepped down the Risperdal, I was able to interject my comments when socializing with strangers—but I became ill and had a mild psychotic episode when I reached the 4 mg level. I would not stray from the house and kept to myself for about a month. That is when my father and Nancy suggested to me that I was sick. After being in denial for about another month, I agreed and had my Risperdal increased to 5 mg upon the recommendation of my psychiatrist.

I was more active and could socialize better with the 5 mg, but I was feeling a little paranoid and fearful. I just learned to live with these negative symptoms, as they were not noticeable to me because my condition was improving in other areas. After four years of university, the negative symptoms gradually increased, and when I graduated, I had to have the Risperdal increased to 6 mg. My brother was the one who noticed that I was not myself and suggested having my medication increased. At that point, I did not care about the adjustment. I just wanted to live without fear and paranoia and wanted to be healthy. I stayed on 6 mg of Risperdal from 2011 to 2012 and finally made the decision to change medications when I discovered that Abilify was available in Canada and, shortly thereafter, was covered by the provincial government's disability drug plan.

From 2012 to 2013, I took 15 mg of Abilify and weaned myself off Risperdal. In the beginning, while I was on 15 mg of Abilify and 6 mg of Risperdal for about a month, I was very active and was always outside visiting friends and riding my electric bike. I would get up in the morning, quickly get ready, be out of the house within the hour, and come home only to sleep. This was a big change compared to always lying around in my bed, full of anxiety and worry, and completely lacking motivation. It helped also that it was summertime where the weather was great and that gave me energy. I would take 15 mg of Abilify in the mornings and 6 mg of Risperdal at bedtime. The reduction of Risperdal would be 0.5 mg every month, and this reduction plan was a rocky one. Many times I would have to increase my Risperdal by 1 mg when I reached the 4 mg level, and a couple times when I reached the 2 mg level.

After one month, in the middle of transitioning between drugs, I could not sleep at night. I was experiencing something like insomnia. I would stay up all night talking to an old friend. Then my psychiatrist prescribed me some lorazepam, which would help me get to sleep, but I discovered it was very addictive, and the withdrawal symptoms were hard on me because a person is not supposed to take it for more than three or four days in a row. I was experiencing stress from Risperdal withdrawal, and at the same time, Abilify was not forceful enough to take care of business on its own (though it seemed to work at times). I did not know what I was going through because it was all new to me, so I stuck it out for a year and ended up in the mental health ward at Peterborough Regional Health Centre when I eliminated Risperdal from my system.

From 2013 to the present, I have been taking 180 mg of Zeldox and 1 mg of Risperdal. Getting off Abilify was depressing because Abilify boosts your mood. It's also used for many forms of depression. It did not help either that it was winter when I stopped taking Abilify; the season also contributed to my low mood. In the beginning, Zeldox made me feel very drowsy. I would take 60 mg of Zeldox with breakfast and 120 mg with dinner, and 1 mg of Risperdal at bedtime. The morning dose didn't make me so drowsy, but after taking my dinner dose of Zeldox, I was wiped out and would crash and need to lie down. I would go to sleep shortly thereafter, barely having enough energy to take my Risperdal. I would go to sleep around 7:00 p.m., wake up around 3:00 a.m., and have a two-hour nap during the day.

As a result, I had the Zeldox reduced to 40 mg in the morning and the same 120 mg at dinnertime. I felt less drowsy on the lowered dose of Zeldox, but this reduction did not fully work in combating my paranoia and fears. I would feel suspicious when running into people in the building if I tried to leave my apartment during one of these fearful episodes. My psychiatrist recommended adding 1 mg more of Risperdal, making it 2 mg at bedtime. I felt better but began losing my motivation, became constipated, and felt hungover in the morning, so I went back to my original dose. After a month of being on 160 mg of Zeldox and 2 mg of Risperdal, I switched to 180 mg of Zeldox and 1 mg of Risperdal. I feel great now, but I try to have dinner later in the evening so that when I do take my 120 mg of Zeldox, I am pretty much settled in for the night.

The pain that you create now is always some form of non-acceptance, some form of unconscious resistance to what is. On the level of thought, the resistance is some form of judgment. On the emotional level, it is some form of negativity. The intensity of the pain depends on the degree of resistance to the present moment, and this in turn depends on how strongly you are identified with your mind.
—Eckhart Tolle, *The Power of Now*

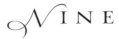

I N E

Spirituality

Eckhart Tolle

One day in 2008, I turned on the television to find Eckhart Tolle on *The Oprah Winfrey Show*. My whole perspective changed when I read *The Power of Now* and, shortly after, *A New Earth*. He talked about how most people are not aware of the feelings or thoughts they experience, and that people often believe, follow, react, and fashion an identity for themselves out of their thought patterns.

When I read or listened to Tolle, I became more aware of myself, and that the negative thoughts and fearful emotions I was experiencing were very common, shared by millions of people across the globe as the human condition. I so strongly identified with my mind, that my dysfunctional thoughts and emotions had taken possession over me. Tolle instructed me to detach myself from them, not to take them literally, and to lighten up.

Tolle says that everyone has an ego, and it should be everyone's goal to get rid of it. The ego is the culprit that can make you feel threatened by others or fearful for no reason. It makes you believe that you are a separate entity from another human being, when in actuality we are all connected through spirit. It makes you believe that others are obstacles in your path when, in fact, they're put in your life to help make you more aware of yourself. Others are not here to make you happy; they are here to present obstacles that you must overcome to move forward with your life.

I found that I was always fearful of others, seeing them as threats. When I realized the way I was feeling was not the fault of others, I began to heal. Every person seems difficult and unique when you are struggling with schizophrenia, and I discovered that no matter how others responded to me, that they were not trying to hurt me. Rather, they were trying to wake me up to reality. I realized that the more I focused on the fact that the people in my life are here to help me, the more I was able to move on to better company. By seeing others as opportunities to build psychological strength, emotional well-being, and spiritual connectedness to God, I was able to keep the right perspective through the adversity often created by the hands of others.

If someone attacks you emotionally or insults you, you should not rush to defend yourself. You will feel hurt and small, but your ego will get smaller and smaller because you do not feed it anymore. Tolle states that you can't be angry with other people just because they are at a different level of awareness; but he also states that others are just reflections of your inner state. And when you clean up your inner pollution, the outside world will be friendly and respond positively.

Tolle states the ego has a shadow within your spirit called the "pain body." This is a trapped negative energy field that you feel when you are resisting reality because it is undesirable to you. He instructs that in order to be free and live in the present moment, you must accept whatever happens or does not happen in that moment.

Tolle also states that most people are either trapped in the past or they are trying to fulfill themselves in some future moment. Both forms of dysfunction sacrifice the present. And many people are caught between desiring and fearing the future at the same time, which creates a lot of anxiety and worry. He states that the more you enter into the present, the more you dissolve your pain body and the higher frequency you will vibrate to, thereby attracting new people and experiences in your life.

For so long, I was not living in the present moment, as I kept reviewing my past, while at the same time dreaming about some future moment where I would complete myself. I was not living and desired a better life. I lived in a constant state of anxiety and worry, fearing that I would not be able to handle the challenges that would be presented to me along the way. Being aware of my dysfunction was not enough to correct it; I had to enter the present moment as much as I could by letting go of the need for control to improve my health and life circumstances. When I began the process of surrender to God, I began to have opportunities with situations and individuals that satisfied my hunger for improvement in my life and health. I realized that I have found forgiveness for the past, as it no longer defines who I am. And it does not matter what the future brings me, because I am content with living in the present moment.

Tolle says that there are very few people chosen to carry the burden of a heavy pain body. Those in this situation, who have been able to process their shadows and release their pasts, do, in fact, become very enlightened individuals. The heaviness of their egos catapults these selected few into higher states of being and understanding as their suffering becomes fuel for consciousness.

The goal, Tolle states, is to quiet the mind and be at peace with yourself and everybody else. If you have glimpses of having no thoughts in your mind, then the path to enlightenment has started, and eventually the present moment will become your dominant state. He also says that the peace you feel has no limits; you just have to tap into it.

This is how you relinquish your fears, by letting go of the need to be in control of others or your environment. This is how true relationships are formed, as you can see another for who he or she really is. He says that true love—a love not known by many people on this earth—is a higher intelligence far greater than what we can comprehend.

The same power that raised Christ from the dead lives on inside of you. The enemy would not be fighting you so hard if he didn't know God had something great in store. I've found the size of your challenge is an indication of the size of your future. If you are facing a big giant challenge, don't be discouraged; that means God has something amazing just up in front of you. He has a new level of your destiny.
—Joel Osteen, *Break Out!*

God

olle got me through some tough times during my early years of recovery, when I was just looking within myself to find answers to what I was going through and why, so I could heal. But I discovered that as much as he helped me out, he also places a lot of the focus of his teachings on the individual being in control of his or her state of mind and spiritual growth. That burden was too much to bear despite the amazing spiritual wisdom and experiences I enjoyed through this false prophet. What I found disturbing was that he did not acknowledge that Jesus is Lord and God, and he said that there are no evil people—just people who are not aware of themselves. Before I was introduced to Tolle, I had a close relationship with Jesus but became disillusioned at the trials and tribulations the Lord was putting me through, and I lost my trust in him. Thankfully I found the Lord again, and regardless of the spiritual and psychological knowledge and wisdom I learned from Tolle, I found that the Lord knows best, and being introduced to Tolle's teachings was just a part of his plan.

When the storms in life come crashing down and there is nowhere to go and no one to turn to for help, that is when you learn to look up. Coming down with schizophrenia was one big storm in my life. I was so overwhelmed that I had no other choice but to seek

God for comfort, guidance, strength, solace, and hope. The valley experiences in life are where you learn the most about yourself and what you are made out of. Recovering from schizophrenia, I had developed a lot of patience, and learned that I can handle an enormous amount of suffering and pain. In order to reach success in life, be on the proper path, and bring glory to God's kingdom, a person must experience the valleys in life. Even though my valley experiences were strenuous, taxing, and exhausting, I knew they were a tool God used to develop my character. Throughout my challenges, I tried my best not to focus on my circumstances, but rather, on what the Lord was trying to teach me and who he wanted me to become.

The storms in life are not meant to be burdens; they are meant to carry you higher in life. Eagles use storms and their winds to soar and fly higher in the air, and that is the Lord's purpose for the storms in our lives, to bring us to a higher place of blessing. I have known, from the moment I was diagnosed with schizophrenia, that God had a purpose other than making me dependent upon him. Unfortunately, many people see the storms in life as obstacles, spend their lives opposing them, and never move on and grow as godly people.

The trials in life are intended to promote a relationship and dialogue with God, and only last as long as they're necessary (and not one second longer) to fulfill God's purpose in you. I know I have developed a close relationship with Jesus because of having schizophrenia, and I still think today, like I always have, that having this mental illness is only temporary. In order to build a large building, construction workers have to dig a deep foundation. The higher the building, the deeper the foundation—just like the trials in life are intended to build the foundation for your character. I do not know what kind of building the Lord is making out of me, but I am aware that it is a big, tall, and strong building because the foundation we have been working on is deep. And I know the Lord has plans for me. When I do reach the mountaintop in life, I won't be blown off the peak, and when I reach heaven, I will take with me who I have become.

God will also use the trials in life to break your individual will and bring you into God's will by removing pride and making you humble. That way God can guide and protect you because he knows what you need in life. When you have to depend upon something higher than yourself to just get by, you lose your pride, and it makes you aware of the suffering of others around you, as pride is a stumbling block to communicating with God.

The devil will throw all kinds of tricks at you to get you to be prideful. Sometimes it is hard to distinguish if God is up to something good in your life because the devil will attack you exactly when God is about to bless you. The devil gets people to mistreat and distract you and tries to throw you off track. Thankfully the Lord intends to turn all things that happen to you into good, and he rewards us double for our trouble.

God is never in a hurry, and he is always on time. He will show you the ways to go. It may take a long time before a door opens or opportunity arises, but it will open if you just stay in faith. God makes you wait because he is developing qualities in you that you will need when the door opens, and whatever is there, you will be equipped for the task at hand. God also works behind the scenes to bring the right people in place and move the wrong people out of your life.

For so long, I thought I could wait for God to bless me, without giving up my individual will and pride. Well, I learned the lesson the hard way: that God can and will outwait you. God works in mysterious ways. He knows the future, so waiting on the Lord is not wasted time. God will turn your ashes into beauty if you let him mold you into the likeness of his son.

CONCLUSION

For the longest time, I could not accept that I have schizophrenia. I was in denial for many years, and it did not help that I had to face being stigmatized by my family and society. I was always thinking of an escape route to freedom from schizophrenia because I was suffering so much, unable to improve my health and quality of life. I was left with no choice but to wait for my mental health to improve and for good things to come my way.

I waited six years to move out of the town I was so dissatisfied with and to talk to someone normal to make a close friendship and attend university. I waited ten years to live on my own after being diagnosed, and almost fourteen years to live life without fear, paranoia, and anxiety. I also waited fourteen years to be able to work full-time and socialize with a group of good people.

Now that I am better and have improved my life, I know what my limits are because I tested them. This has given me confidence and freed up some space for me to maneuver while I keep trying to do better. I know now I am a worthy individual and capable of so much more. This has made me a happy and content person because I have hope. I know the future looks bright, and I will continue to stretch beyond my comfort zone to take on new challenges. I am excited to see what God will do in my life and look forward to keeping you updated. Please feel free to visit my website at davidlachapelle.ca or e-mail me at david@davidlachapelle.ca. I would love to hear from you.

Manufactured by Amazon.ca
Bolton, ON

35298966R00039